GERMS AND DISEASE

HOW DO WE FIGHT GERMS?

By Kathryn Kroe

Cavendish Square
New York

Published in 2023 by Cavendish Square Publishing, LLC
29 East 21st Street, New York, NY 10010

Website: cavendishsq.com

Library of Congress Cataloging-in-Publication Data

Names: Kroe, Kathryn, author.
Title: How do we fight germs? / Kathryn Kroe.
Description: New York : Cavendish Square Publishing, [2023] | Series: Germs and disease | Includes bibliographical references and index.
Identifiers: LCCN 2021055538 | ISBN 9781502665287 (library binding) | ISBN 9781502665270 (paperback) | ISBN 9781502665294 (ebook)
Subjects: LCSH: Immunity—Juvenile literature. | Bacteria—Juvenile literature. | Infection—Juvenile literature.
Classification: LCC QR181.8 .K76 2023 | DDC 616.07/9—dc23/eng/20211208
LC record available at https://lccn.loc.gov/2021055538

Editor: Kathryn Kroe
Copyeditor: Jane Katirgis
Designer: Andrea Davison-Bartolotta

The photographs in this book are used by permission and through the courtesy of: Cover MP kullimratchai/Shutterstock.com; series art backgrounds CHIARA VFX/Shutterstock.com; p. 5 Wirestock Creators/Shutterstock.com; p. 6 txking/Shutterstock.com; p. 8 Natalia Mels/Shutterstock.com; p. 10 Astrid Gast/Shutterstock.com; p. 11 frank60/Shutterstock.com; pp. 12, 21 Everett Collection/Shutterstock.com; p. 14 Gorodenkoff/Shutterstock.com; p. 16 Naci Yavuz/Shutterstock.com; p. 17 Cosmin Manci/Shutterstock.com; p. 19 J J Osuna Caballero/Shutterstock.com; p. 23 Science History Images/Alamy Stock Photo; p. 24 Rattiya Thongdumhyu/Shutterstock.com; p. 26 rumka_vodki/Shutterstock.com; p. 28 Oksana Kuzmina/Shutterstock.com; p. 30 Designua/Shutterstock.com; p. 31 PBXStudio/Shutterstock.com; p. 32 VectorMine/Shutterstock.com; p. 34 DGLimages/Shutterstock.com; p. 37 Ann Rodchua/Shutterstock.com; pp. 38-39 DisobeyArt/Shutterstock.com.

CPSIA compliance information: Batch #CSCSQ23: For further information contact Cavendish Square Publishing LLC, New York, New York, at 1-877-980-4450.

Printed in the United States of America

CONTENTS

INTRODUCTION

In 2020, the World Health Organization (WHO) declared a global **pandemic**. One disease was spreading all over the world, wreaking havoc on people's lives. Living through a pandemic has made most people more aware of germs than ever before. They pay more attention to where germs could be hiding and have taken more measures to reduce their exposure to germs and make it difficult for germs to spread.

This pandemic was caused by a coronavirus—COVID-19. Viruses are one of the more sneaky microorganisms. Microorganisms are organisms so tiny you can only see them with a microscope. Viruses want to get into our bodies and infect us, so they often mutate, or change, to get past our bodies' defense systems. The virus that causes COVID-19 is especially good at that, making it much harder to control and stop the spread of the germ.

"Germ" is a word we have all heard for as long as we can remember, but what are germs? How does the body know how to fight them? How can we keep ourselves healthy?

Throughout history, we have learned from our mistakes and triumphs in our war against some microorganisms that make us sick. Especially now, when germs are making such a big impact on everyday life, it's important to understand germs and diseases they cause so we can be prepared to fight them.

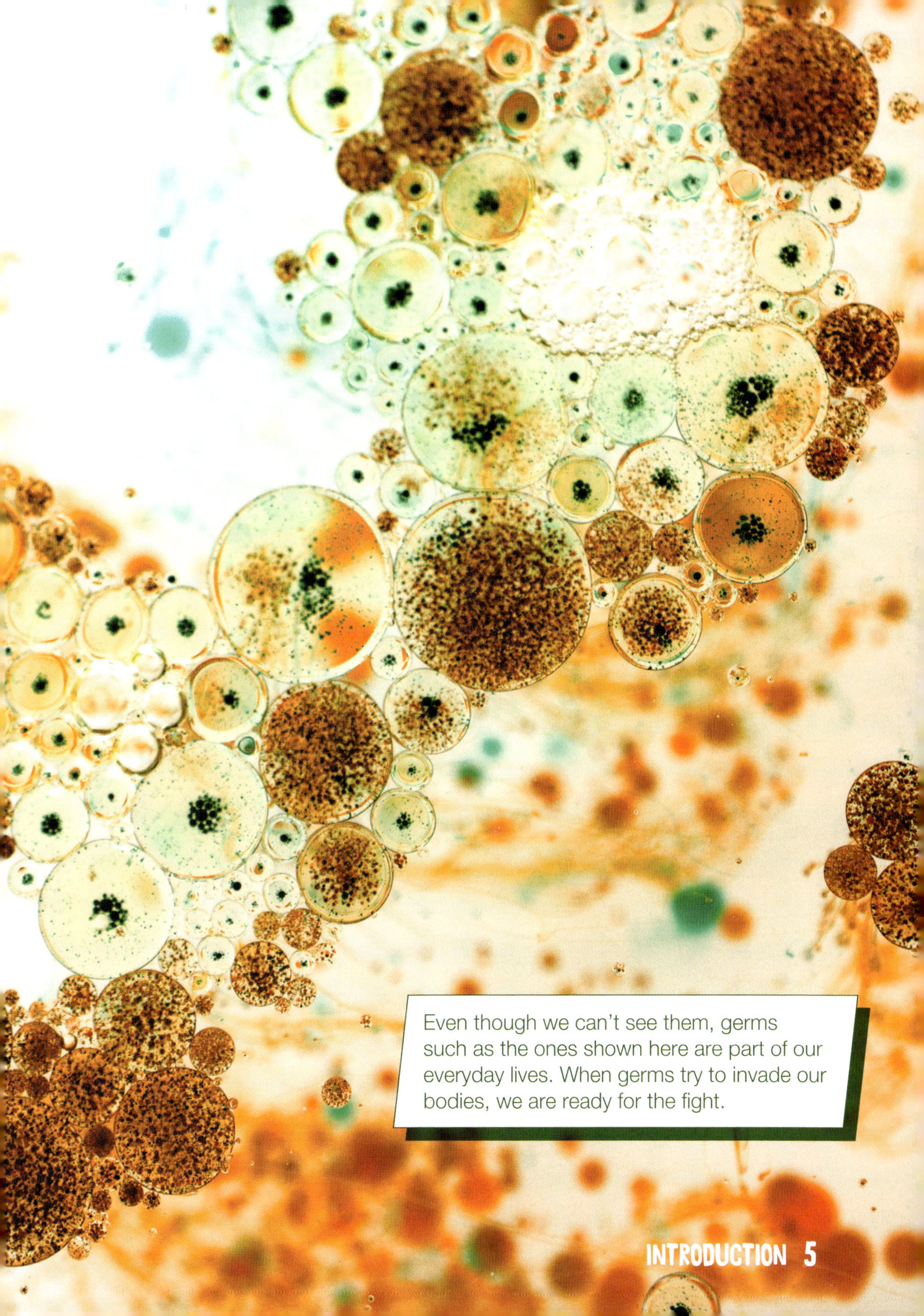

Even though we can't see them, germs such as the ones shown here are part of our everyday lives. When germs try to invade our bodies, we are ready for the fight.

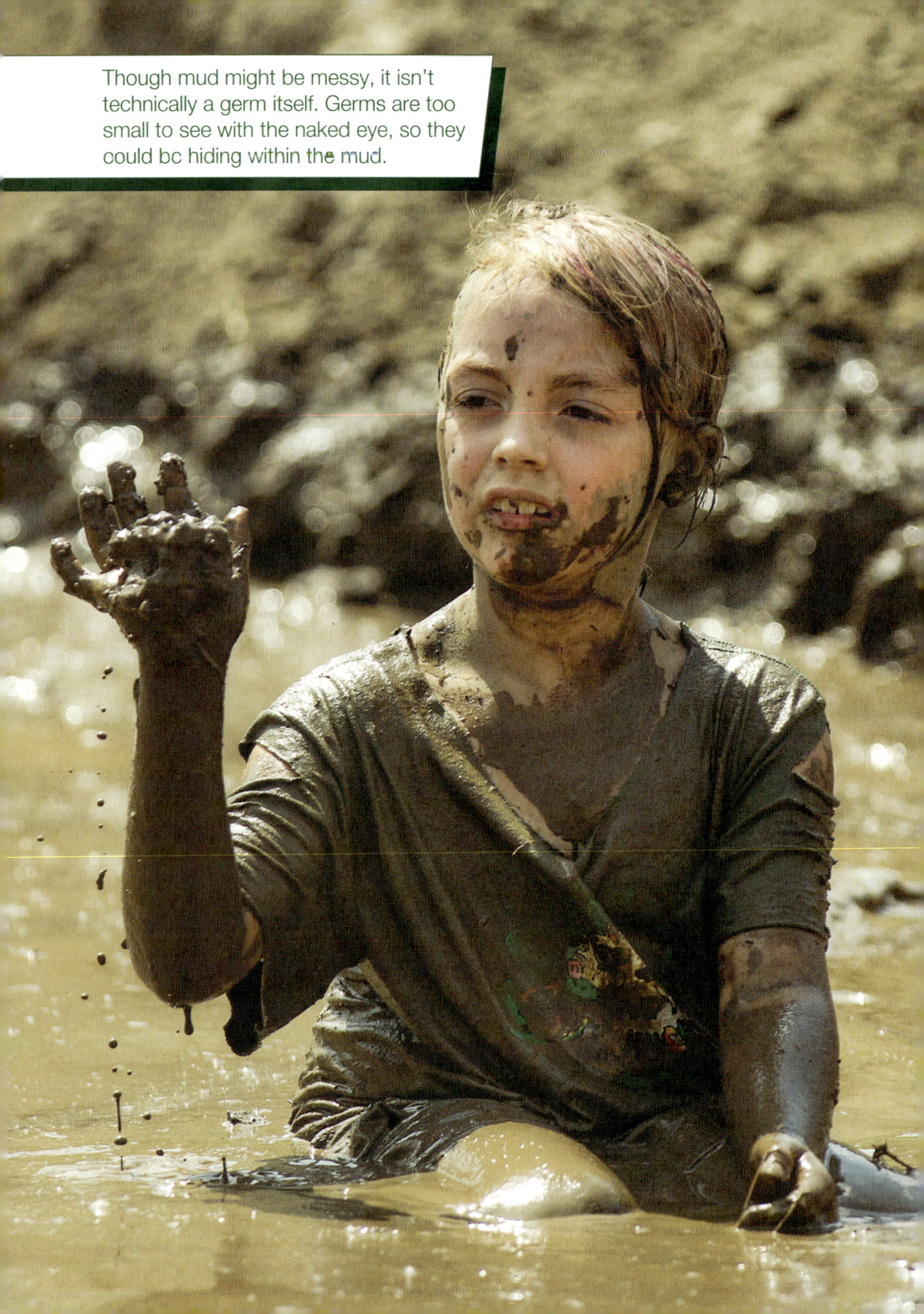

Though mud might be messy, it isn't technically a germ itself. Germs are too small to see with the naked eye, so they could be hiding within the mud.

CHAPTER 1

WHAT ARE GERMS?

Bugs, mud, and other slimy, gooey things are often mistaken for germs by young children. However, these substances are not actually germs, though they may carry these microorganisms.

Microbes, such as bacteria and some kinds of fungi, are so small that we can't see them without a microscope. Many microbes are helpful to our bodies and the environment, but some microbes cause disease. These microbes are called germs. The term "germ" describes four main groups of tiny organisms—bacteria, viruses, fungi, and protozoa—that can cause infectious diseases. Germs can sneak into our bodies in lots of different ways. Some germs that cause only mild sickness can help our bodies' defense systems become stronger. When other germs enter our body, they can cause serious symptoms because our body is being attacked.

BACTERIA

Bacteria are very small, single-celled organisms. Most bacteria aren't harmful to humans. In actuality, many types of bacteria are required to keep us healthy. Some of these good bacteria keep bad bacteria out. We also use bacteria in some foods. Have you ever eaten yogurt or cheese? If you have, you've eaten healthy bacteria.

FUNGI

When you hear the word "fungus," you may think of moldy bread. There are many varieties of fungi. We even eat several forms, such as mushrooms, some cheeses, and yeast. Fungi have also helped us treat other diseases.

However, some fungi can cause illness in humans. Examples include skin conditions such as athlete's foot or infections caused

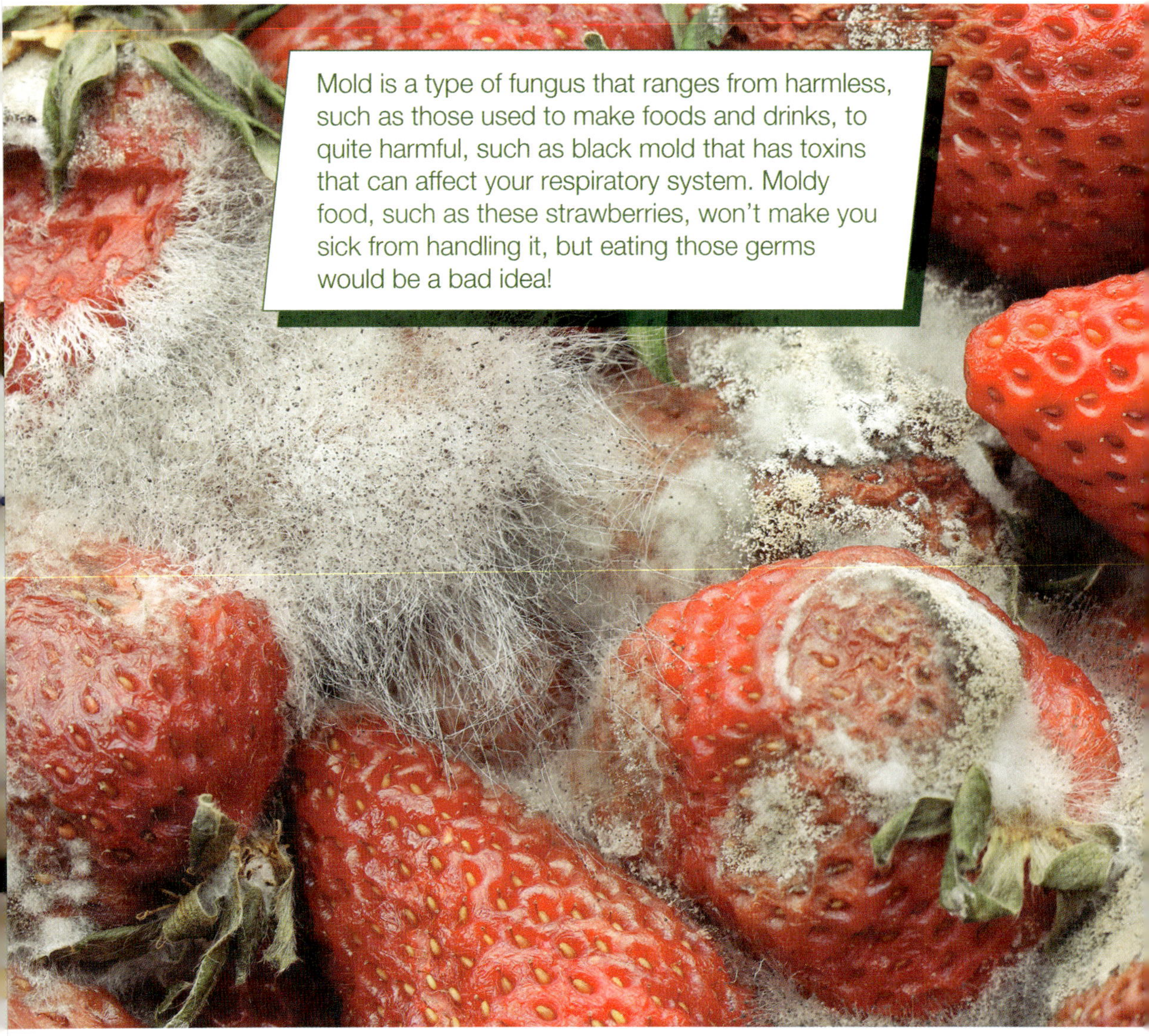

Mold is a type of fungus that ranges from harmless, such as those used to make foods and drinks, to quite harmful, such as black mold that has toxins that can affect your respiratory system. Moldy food, such as these strawberries, won't make you sick from handling it, but eating those germs would be a bad idea!

by yeast in the body. Usually, fungal infections are easily treatable, but for some people with weakened immune systems, they can be dangerous.

Protozoa

Protozoa are one-celled organisms, much like bacteria. They often live outside of humans in things such as food, water, and insects.

We all know mosquitoes as the pests that leave itchy welts on our skin, but did you know they can carry germs? Mosquitoes in some parts of the world carry a dangerous protozoan that can cause malaria, a disease that can lead to chills, fever, sweating, and sometimes death.

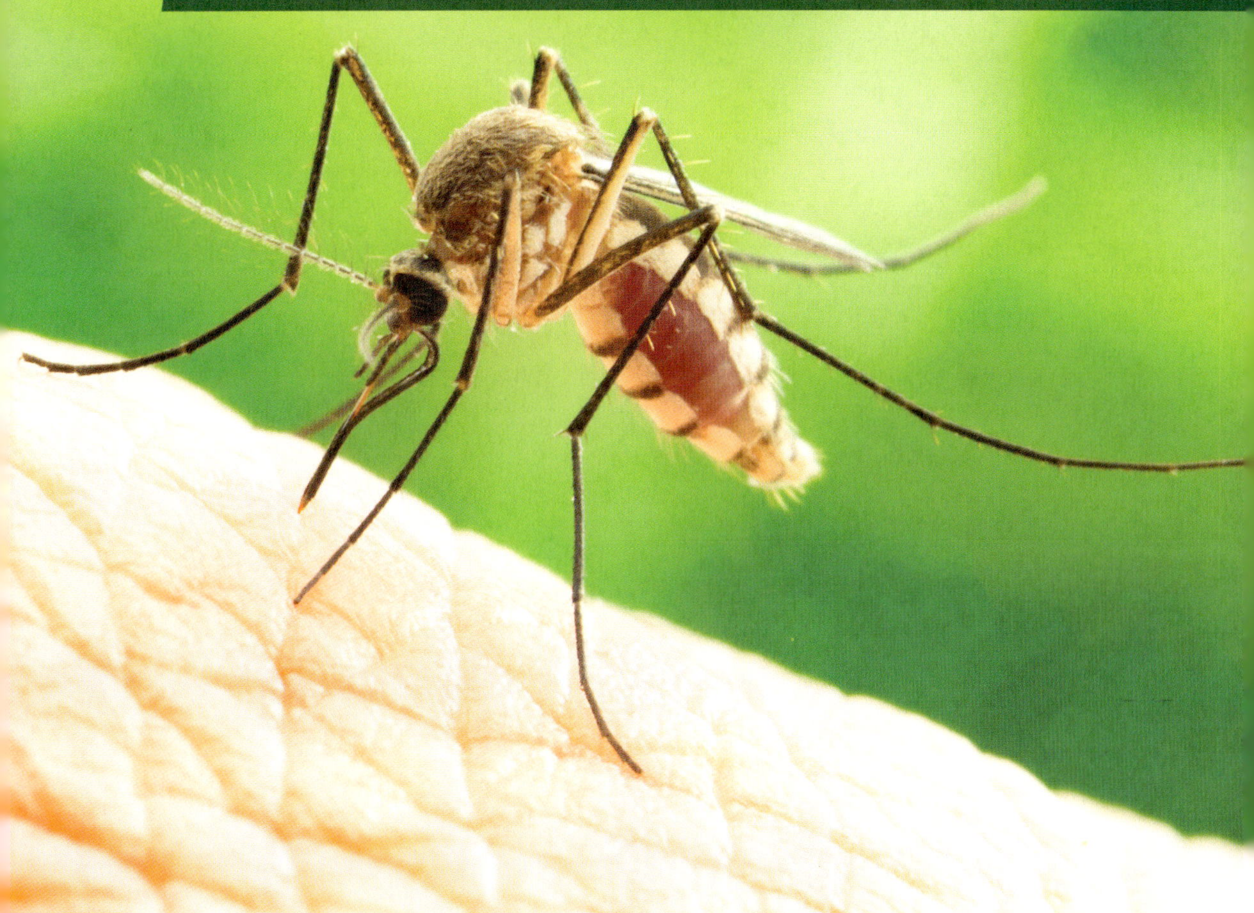

DANGEROUS GERMS THROUGHOUT HISTORY AND TODAY

Over the centuries, dangerous germs have killed millions of people. The Spanish flu was a deadly virus. More people died in the Spanish flu pandemic of 1918, which took place during World War I (1914–1918), than were killed in battle in that war.

The Black Death, which is one of the names for a deadly pandemic in the 14th century, was caused by contagious bacteria and killed more than one-fourth of the population of Europe at the time. Smallpox and other illnesses brought to the Americas by European colonizers devastated indigenous populations.

In the 1980s, AIDS was first identified, and it has claimed an estimated 36 million lives since then. HIV, the virus that causes AIDS, is now treatable. As medicine continues to advance, HIV infections and AIDS may soon be curable.

Dangerous germs continue to affect us today. As of January 2022, the COVID-19 pandemic had infected more than 335,000,000 people worldwide with more than 5 million deaths.

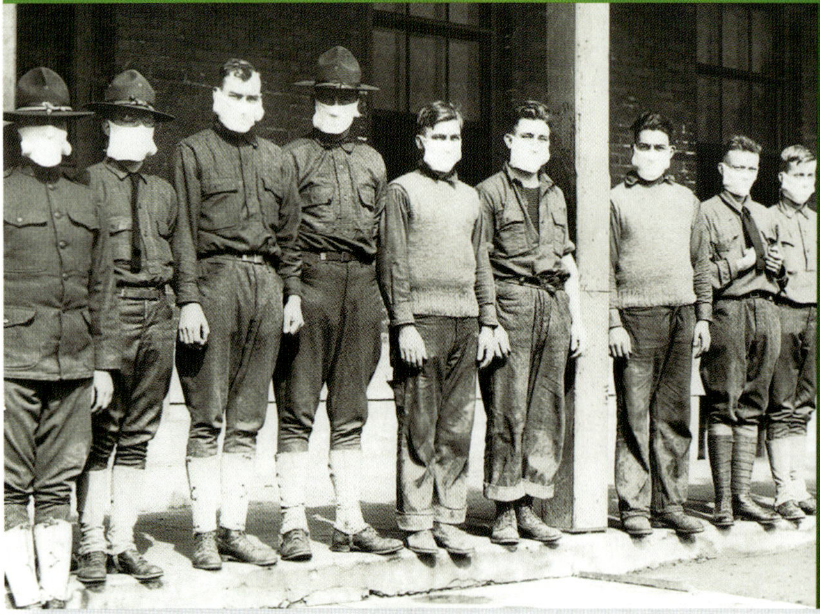

In 1918 during the Spanish flu pandemic, doctors and scientists didn't understand germs well or have the resources we have today. Still, they had the idea that masks could help slow the spread of the dangerous germ.

If harmful protozoa invade your body, they can cause diseases such as malaria.

Understanding different types of germs helps us understand how to protect ourselves from them. Microbes are always changing and evolving to try to sneak past our defenses. However, science and medicine also constantly evolve to try to keep us one step ahead of the germs.

WHAT DO YOU THINK?

1. Why do we use things such as dirt to explain germs to children?
2. Why do you think we focus our resources on fighting some germs more than others?
3. Do you think there are any similarities between the COVID-19 pandemic and other pandemics throughout history?

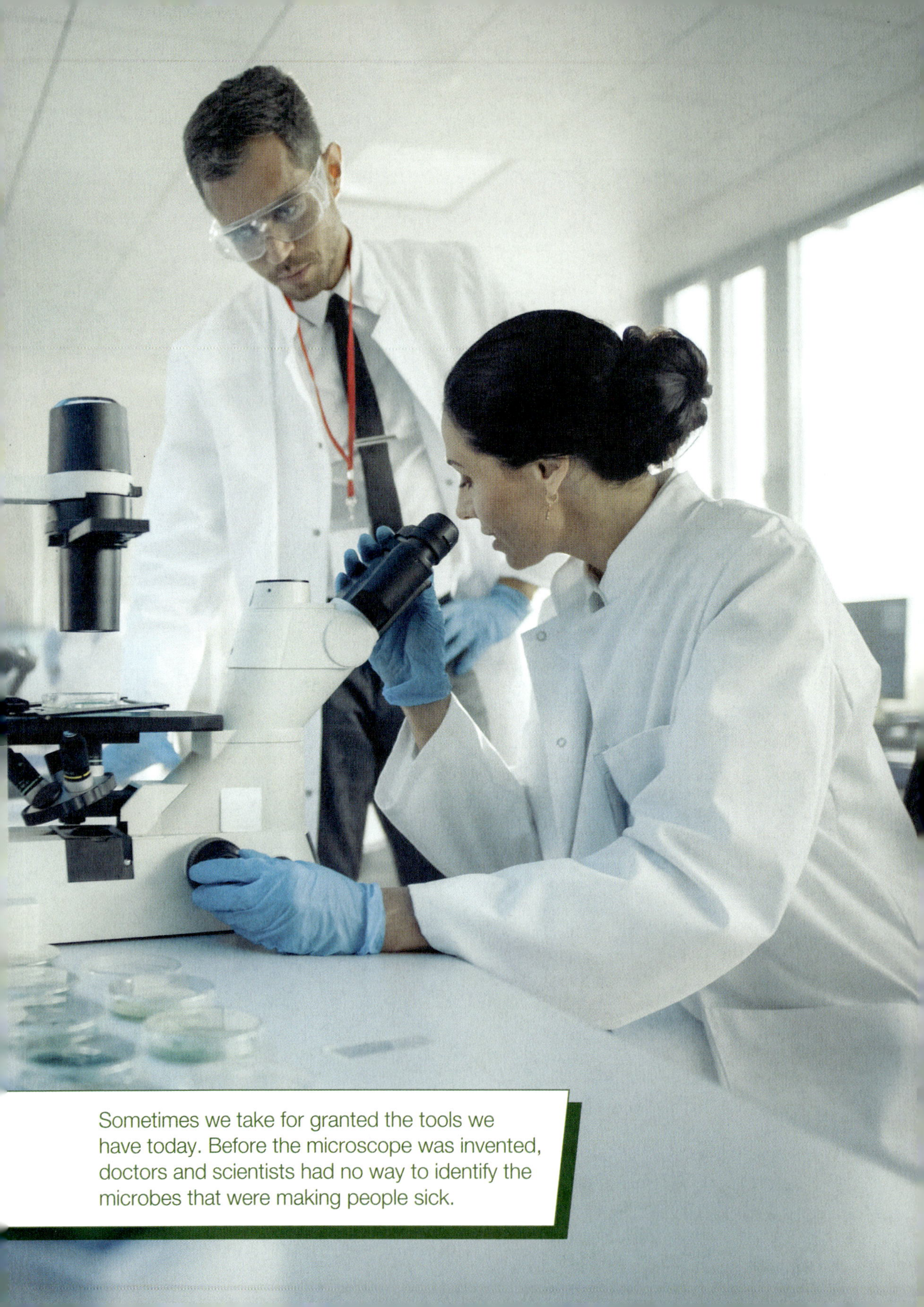

Sometimes we take for granted the tools we have today. Before the microscope was invented, doctors and scientists had no way to identify the microbes that were making people sick.

CHAPTER 2

HOW HAVE MEDICINE AND SCIENCE EVOLVED?

Today, we have a strong understanding of germs. We can see them with microscopes and identify them with testing tools to figure out which microbes are making us sick. However, it is only recently in human history that we have developed these tools and gained a true understanding, rather than an educated guess, of what is happening to our bodies. The microscope was invented at the end of the 16th century. Before that, doctors and scientists could identify the effects of germs and disease and attempt to treat patients through trial and error, but they didn't have the tools to have a true understanding of what was causing the disease or infection. Medicine and **epidemiology** have made strides to achieve what we know today.

THEORIES THROUGHOUT HISTORY

When we get sick, it can be scary. However, we usually understand why we feel sick or can consult medical professionals to help us understand and treat our condition. Throughout history, germs still caused the same issues we see today, but there was often minimal understanding about what was going on. Because people wanted to understand the why and how, many different and often inaccurate things were theorized as causing or curing illness. Still, some of these things led to later breakthroughs in medicine.

In ancient Mesopotamia and ancient Egypt, doctors thought supernatural forces were to blame for disease. There were different classes of disease-treating professionals in both civilizations. There would be someone who specialized in the spells and rituals they thought necessary to cure people, and other practitioners to treat symptoms. These practitioners did use some remedies that still have merit today. They knew about the need to wash a wound, keep it clean, and apply clean bandages. They also discovered natural ingredients such as garlic, oil of fir, and honey that had **antiseptic** and antibiotic properties.

The ancient Greek doctor Hippocrates, often called the Father of Medicine, was the first to state that disease had nothing to do with gods or evil spirits. He separated medicine from religion. However, his main theory about the human body was incorrect. He said it had four "**humors**," black bile, yellow bile, phlegm, and blood, and stated that illness occurred when one of these humors was out of balance. Hippocrates did stress the importance of fresh

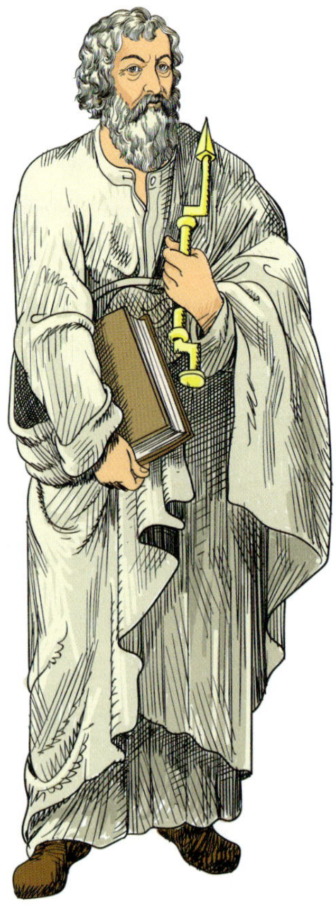

Hippocrates's impact on medicine is still felt today. In fact, modern doctors still swear a version of the Hippocratic oath, promising to do no harm to patients.

air, a good diet, and plenty of exercise to help the body heal itself. Hippocrates's students had to swear an oath to help their patients and do no harm before they could treat the sick.

During the Middle Ages, Persian doctor Abu Bakr Muhammad ibn Zakariya al-Razi, commonly known as al-Razi, observed his hospital patients carefully and took precise notes. These observations led him to discover the difference between measles and smallpox. Another famous Persian doctor, Abu Ali al-Husain ibn Sina, commonly known as Avicenna, stressed the need for cleanliness during surgery to keep open wounds from becoming infected. Through observation, these men were able to identify and use information they couldn't fully comprehend.

Breakthroughs in Understanding

In Italy during the Renaissance, Girolamo Fracastoro was a multitalented man: a doctor, astronomer, philosopher, and poet. He theorized that infection was caused by "seeds of disease" that multiplied within the body and spread through human breathing. At the time, there was no way to prove his theory correct. Athanasius Kircher was a German writer and scientist who wrote a **treatise** on an epidemic of **bubonic plague** that hit Italy in 1656. In it, he stated that tiny animals might

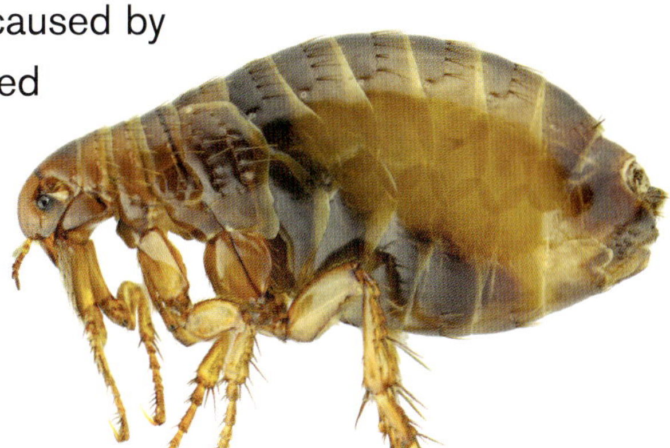

Athanasius Kircher's theory that bubonic plague was spread by tiny animals would eventually be proven correct. Fleas, such as this one, that travel on small rodents were shown to transmit the disease.

SPIRITUAL MEDICINE TODAY

As understanding of germs and disease increased, more medical professionals agreed with Hippocrates that disease and spiritual well-being were separate. However, some medical professionals in different parts of the world still believe there is an important connection between health and spiritual life force.

Practitioners of traditional Chinese medicine (TCM) have existed for thousands of years and believe that a spiritual life force called Qi needs to be in balance to keep people healthy. If Qi is imbalanced, it is thought that it will cause illness and disease. Qi is made up of **complementary** forces, yin and yang, and an alteration of one is thought to be the underlying cause of some diseases.

To treat an imbalance, and such an illness or disease, practitioners of TCM believe you must balance internal body organs with Earth's external elements. This may sound far-fetched to people who have grown up with medicine that has no spiritual component, but most people are actually familiar with several common TCM treatments. These include acupuncture, massage, cupping, herbal remedies, and tai chi. Western medicine, based strictly on science, agrees that some of these TCM treatments may have merit when combined with Western ways to treat disease. Western medicine practitioners feel that TCM should not be used in place of science-based treatment for serious conditions but could be beneficial as a complementary treatment by a certified professional.

have caused the disease. These doctors and scientists were on the right track, even before tools were developed to help research their ideas.

It was Antonie van Leeuwenhoek of Holland, however, who made the most significant discoveries about disease during this era.

While working as a fabric merchant, he learned how to grind lenses for glasses and then taught himself how to make simple microscopes. He designed and built more than 500 microscopes during his life. He became so skilled that some of his creations magnified small items more than 200 times. Using these tools, he discovered bacteria, parasites, blood cells, and many other microscopic things. His research findings were widely circulated and opened up a new world of microscopic life to scientists. Now that they had the tools with which to identify their microscopic enemies, scientists could actually begin to find ways to combat the germs that caused disease.

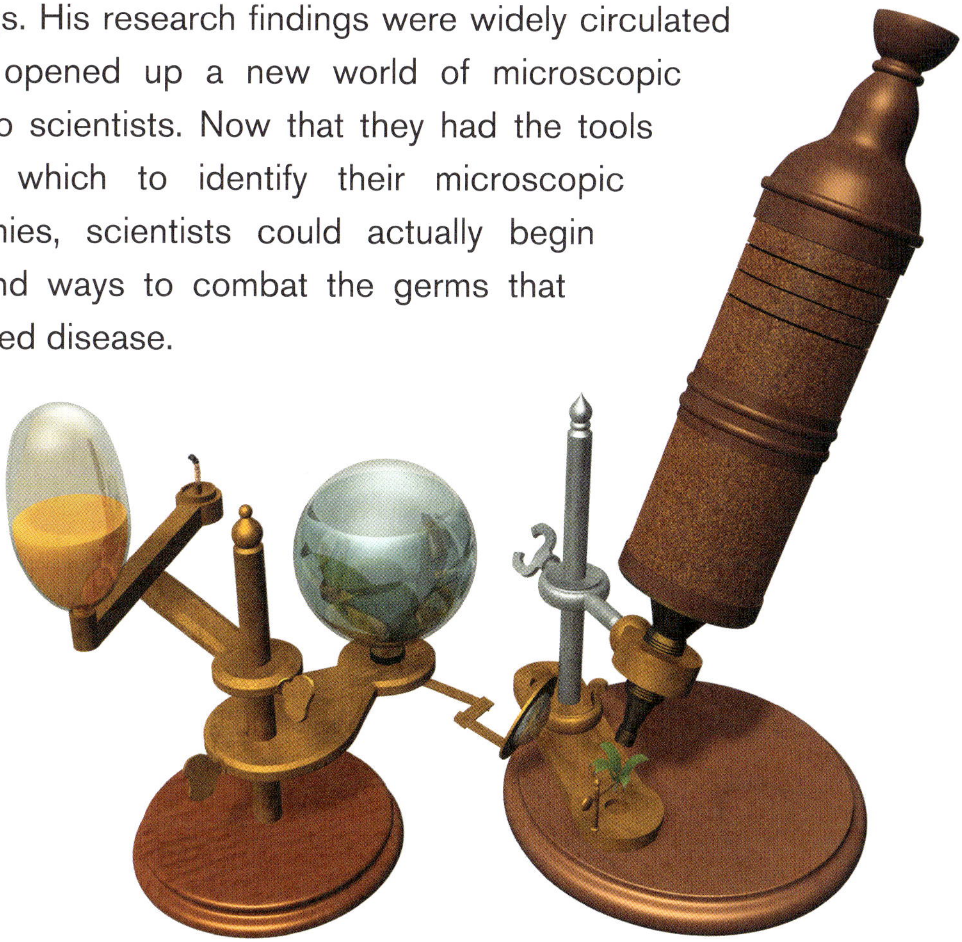

Though they may not look the same as they do today, early microscopes were groundbreaking. Once the technology was invented, it would only be improved and strengthened over the years.

LOUIS PASTEUR

French scientist Louis Pasteur started his career as a chemist working with the wine industry, but he soon became fascinated with bacteriology, the study of bacteria. Up until that time, scientists still believed in the theory known as spontaneous generation, in which living things, such as germs, could spring up from nonliving things, such as the earth. Pasteur proved that even microscopic creatures could come only from other microscopic creatures. Through his research and experiments, Pasteur figured out how to keep wine, beer, and milk safe through a heating process now called pasteurization. Another of Pasteur's great achievements was showing how diseases are caused by germs that multiply in the body. He built on Edward Jenner's work, learned to weaken germs in a laboratory, and improved vaccination methods. He was able to create a vaccine for rabies, which was previously thought to be an incurable disease.

JOSEPH LISTER

Another scientist, British surgeon Joseph Lister, built on Pasteur's work. For years, people believed that infections were caused solely by bad air. Wound **sepsis**—the term for a wound overcome by infection—was thought to occur when the injured area started to decompose. However, so many patients were dying of this condition that Lister suspected there was something more at work. He did his best to encourage the safe healing of wounds and tried to find a likely cause for these infections. Lister made the connection between germs in the air, from Pasteur's work, and wound sepsis. He knew that carbolic acid had been successfully

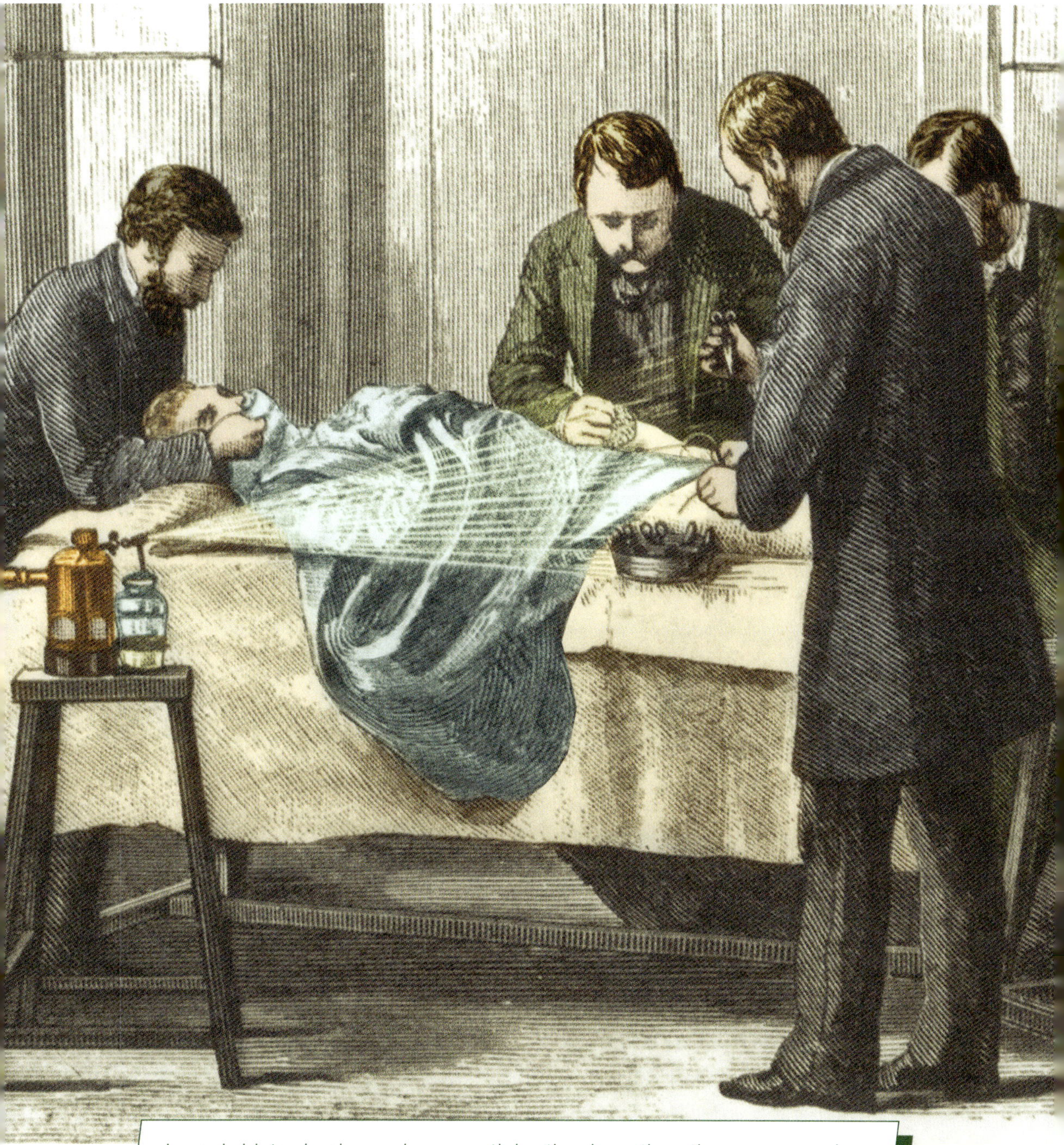

Joseph Lister is shown here participating in antiseptic surgery, using sterilized instruments and conditions. He invited the operation to be witnessed and publicized to prove the success of the technique.

used to rid cattle of a disease-causing parasite, and he started cleaning wounds with a solution of carbolic acid. In 1867, he announced his patients had been free from sepsis for nine months. By the 1870s, German surgeons began practicing what came to be called antiseptic surgery, including using sterilized instruments. On October 26, 1877, Lister carried out an operation under antiseptic conditions and made sure that the operation was both witnessed and well publicized. Antiseptic surgery soon became accepted almost everywhere, nearly eliminating postsurgical infections.

SIR ALEXANDER FLEMING

Sir Alexander Fleming, a British scientist, accidentally discovered the germ-killing power of *Penicillium notatum*, the scientific name

Fleming's discovery was one of the happiest accidents in the history of germ fighting. The culture plate below shows penicillin mold, which grew when he forgot about a culture plate with some bacteria on it. The mold, *Penicillium notatum*, killed all the bacteria around it.

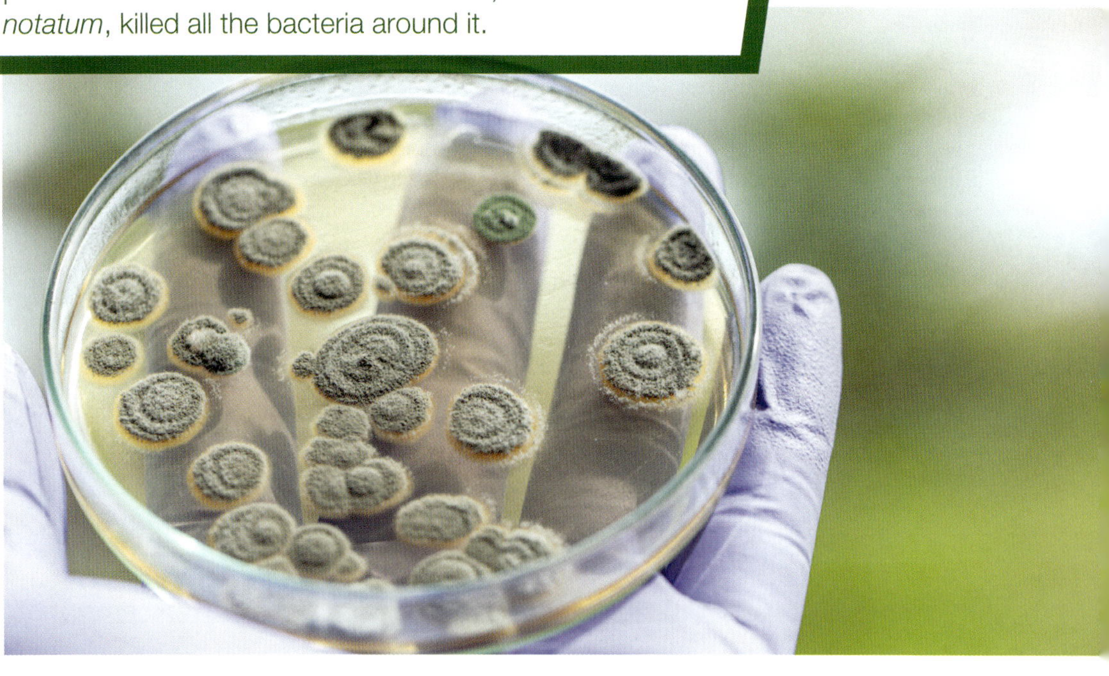

of a mold from which the lifesaving antibiotic penicillin was first created. By chance, he had forgotten about a culture plate he had left with some bacteria on it. When he returned, Fleming was astonished to find that a tiny bit of penicillium mold had sprouted in the plate and killed all the bacteria around it. The discovery would eventually open up a new era for medicine. It was not until 1940, however, that this information was fully embraced. Two British scientists, Howard Florey and Ernst Chain, found that penicillin protected mice against a number of bacteria. This jump-started the development of penicillin for human use. It had a huge impact in saving soldiers' lives during World War II (1939–1945). Fleming, Florey, and Chain won the 1945 Nobel Prize in medicine for their discovery. Penicillin was available for general public use by the end of the decade. This led to research on other forms of antibiotics.

These breakthroughs were all critical to getting where we are today in treating and identifying disease. We will only continue to make groundbreaking discoveries going forward as we further our understanding of both germs and the human body.

WHAT DO YOU THINK?

1. How do you think some doctors came up with theories so close to the truth without the tools to prove them?
2. Which scientist's discovery do you think played the biggest part in the fight against germs?
3. Why are people doubtful of new medical breakthroughs?

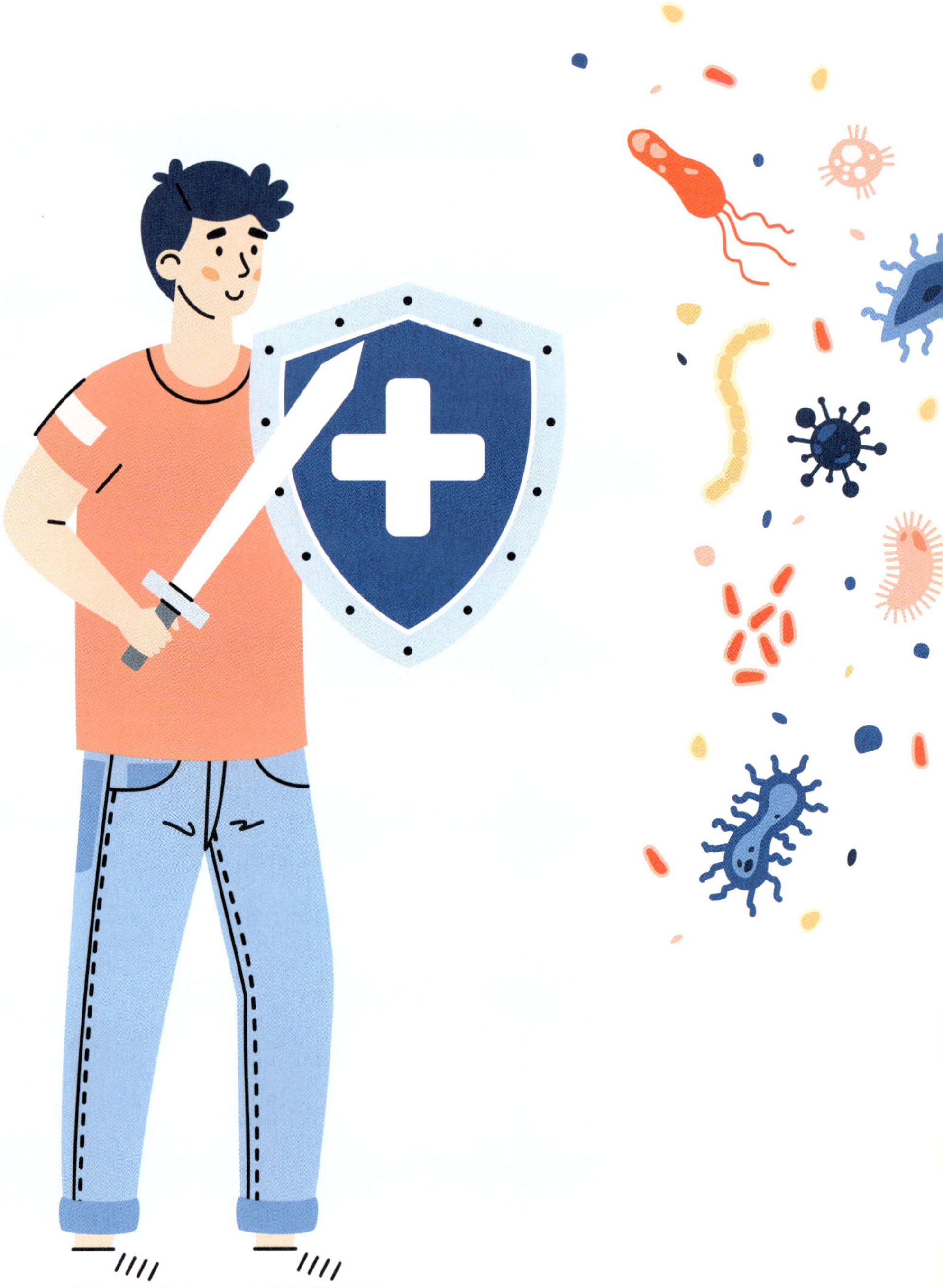

While people with shields can't protect us from germs, our white blood cells work hard every day like warriors to keep us healthy.

CHAPTER 3

HOW DO OUR BODIES PROTECT US?

The good news is that our bodies are ready to fight against harmful germs! This natural defense system is called the immune system, a complicated network of cells and organs that work together. The immune system guards the body against attacks by "foreign" invaders—things it identifies as not belonging in the body. Every cell contains specific molecules that identify it as belonging to the body. The immune system normally doesn't attack any cells that have the right identification.

However, the immune system can and will react to millions of foreign germs. It fights them off by creating special substances and cells called **antibodies**. These antibodies catch and destroy all the outside germs. The body also has immune organs in it. These are called lymphoid organs because they create and send out **lymphocytes**, a type of white blood cell. White blood cells are considered the "warriors" of the immune system.

INNATE IMMUNITY

Though the immune system does get stronger with time, we all have an innate immunity at birth. It provides general, or nonspecific, defense against germs. It continues to be the first response to foreign invaders throughout our lives. Even our skin is part of our

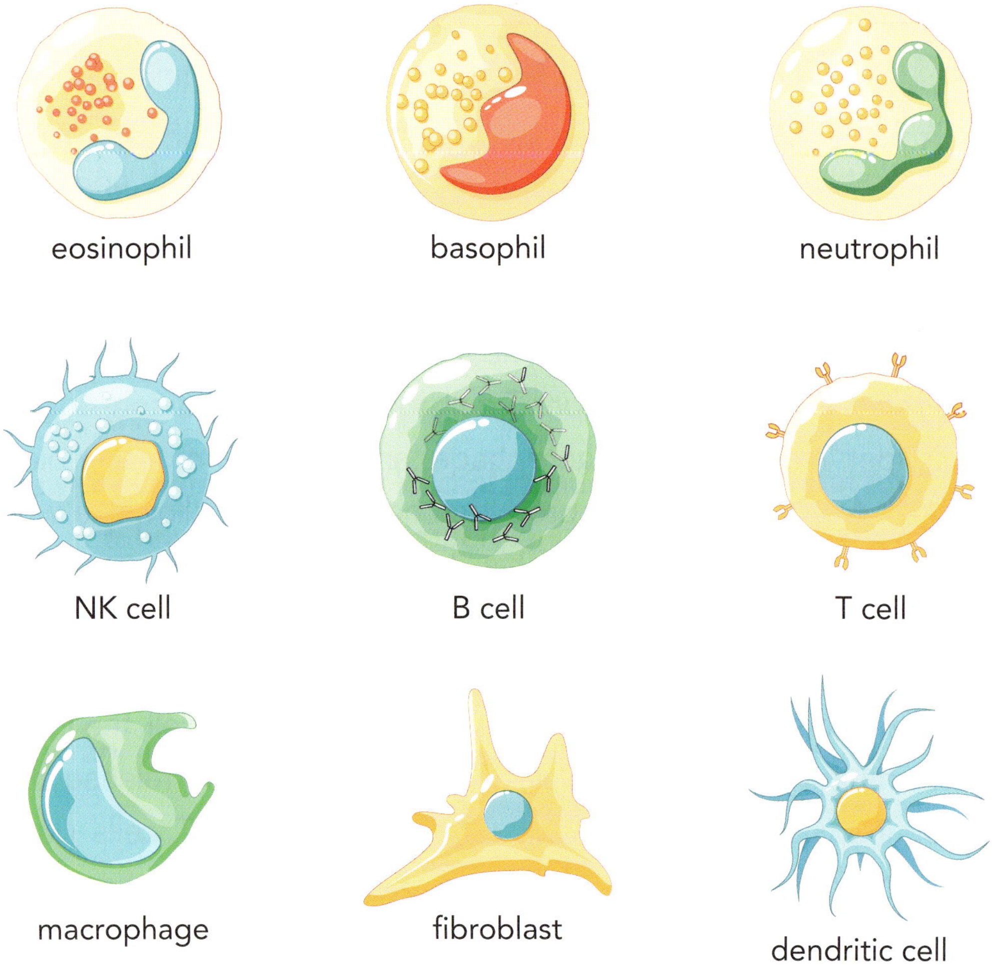

Some examples of the key cells in the immune system are shown here. Each immune system cell knows its job. They all work together to stop the foreign invader from continuing to make your body sick.

ORGANS OF THE IMMUNE SYSTEM

Various organs in the body have a role in making our defense system work correctly. Our skin and the **mucous membranes** in our nose and throat act as the first line of defense. They are physical barriers to prevent harmful germs from entering the body at all. Coughing and sneezing are also responses in attempt to prevent foreign invaders.

About the Author

Kathryn Kroe has a master's degree in public health from the University at Buffalo and a bachelor's degree in education from SUNY Buffalo State College. She is passionate about spreading accurate information and helping young people understand issues pertaining to their health and the health of those around them. She currently lives in Lockport, New York, with her husband and two toddlers. She enjoys walking with her family, playing with her Australian shepherd, Zoey, and traveling to see new places.

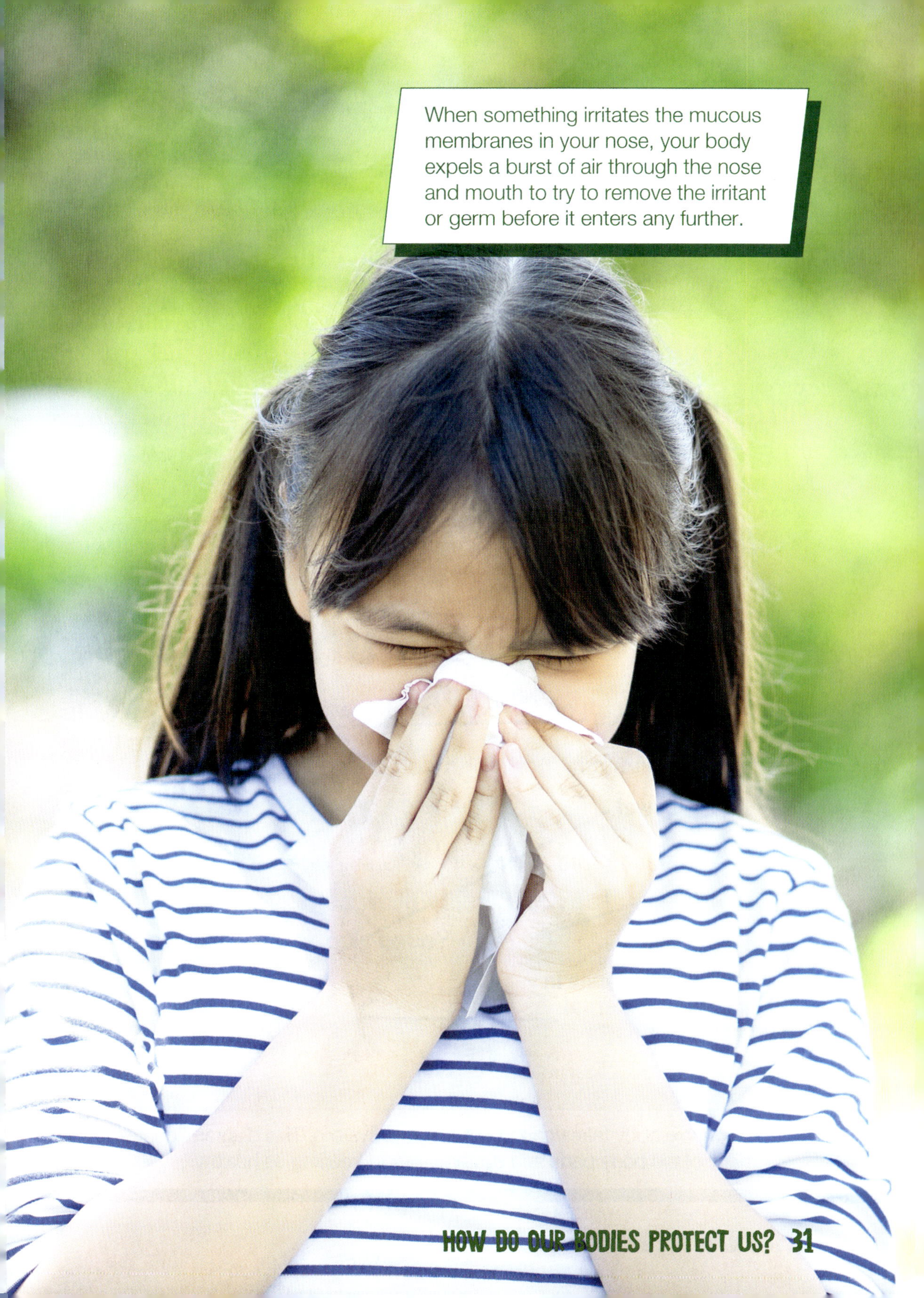

When something irritates the mucous membranes in your nose, your body expels a burst of air through the nose and mouth to try to remove the irritant or germ before it enters any further.

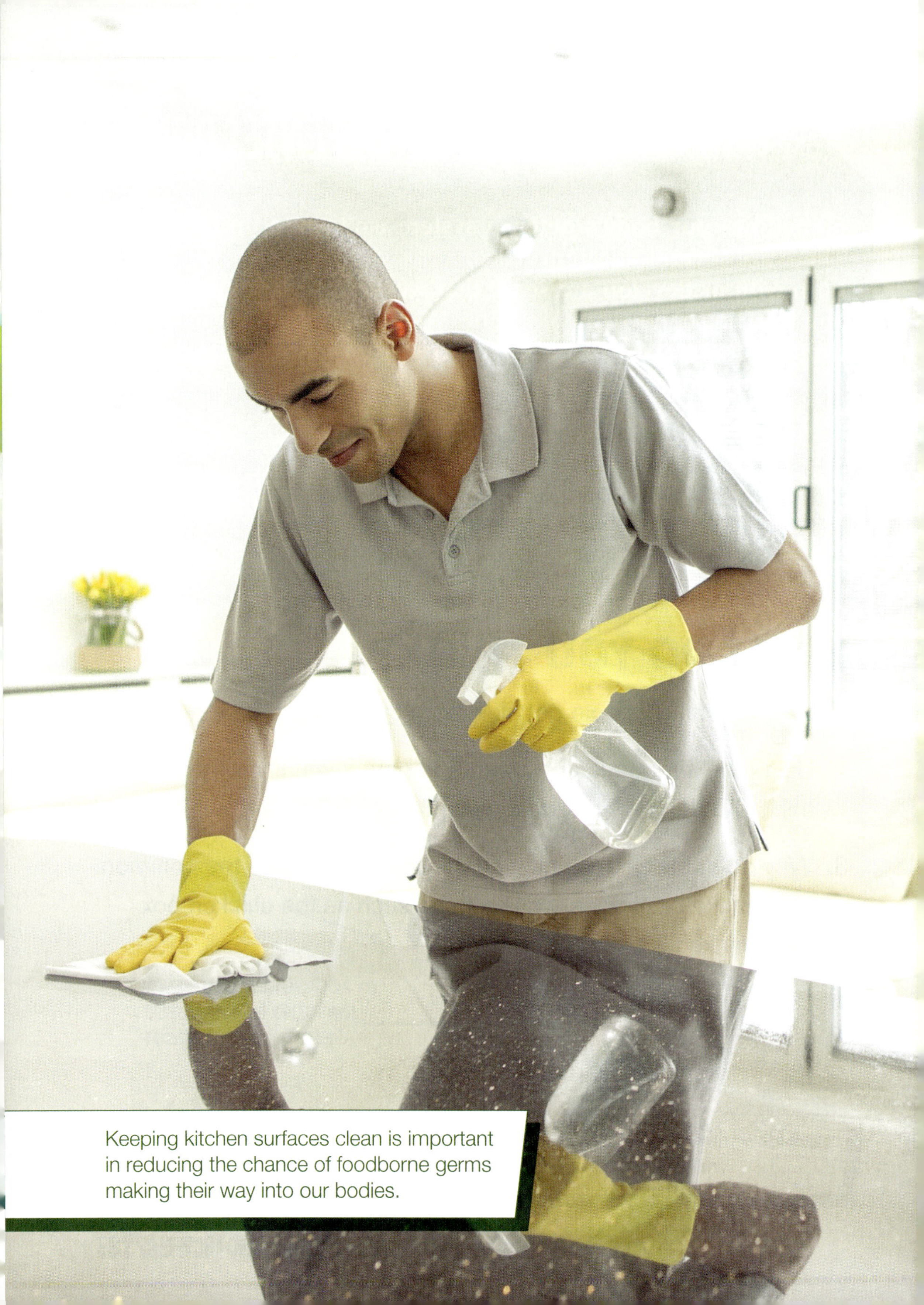

Keeping kitchen surfaces clean is important in reducing the chance of foodborne germs making their way into our bodies.

CHAPTER 4

WHAT CAN WE DO TO PROTECT OURSELVES?

Today, with our understanding of germs, there are many different ways we know we can protect ourselves to prevent our bodies from having to fight invaders in the first place. There are some basic precautions to defend against germs. These range from simple, everyday precautions to vaccines and following public health recommendations.

Keeping Clean

Your chance of catching illnesses through casual contact is greatly reduced if you wash your hands regularly with soap and warm water. Properly handling and preparing food also helps. Keeping kitchen counters, cutting boards, knives, and other utensils clean, especially before and after use, reduces the chances of spreading foodborne illnesses. So does properly refrigerating and freezing foods and keeping certain foods separate from others—such as making sure raw poultry and other meats do not potentially contaminate vegetables or other foods. Even just covering your mouth when you sneeze or cough helps when it comes to mitigating the risk of spreading airborne bacterial and viral infections.

Disinfectants are also helpful. A disinfectant is a substance that destroys germs on nonliving things, such as clothes or floors.

Disinfectants are added to a city's sewage system to keep it from spreading dangerous germs. They also are used in hospitals. At home, though, household disinfectants are usually so mild that plain soap and water are just as useful. There are several basic types of disinfectants. These include the following:

- isopropyl (rubbing) alcohol, used to disinfect items such as thermometers
- formaldehyde, used by hospitals to disinfect equipment
- hypochlorites, including chlorine bleach, found in household detergents as well as in sewage treatment plants
- iodophors, which contain iodine and are used to disinfect large areas in hospitals
- phenols, used to disinfect floors, garbage cans, and more

Cleaning and disinfecting are especially important to reduce transmission of germs that live on surfaces.

Vaccines

There are also vaccinations to protect us from disease. In the United States, Canada, and other countries, we are vaccinated as very young children against many diseases, such as smallpox, polio, measles, and tetanus.

There are six main types of vaccines:

- live attenuated vaccines: These contain germs that have been altered so they can't cause disease. Some examples of live attenuated vaccines are measles, mumps, and rubella (MMR) and chicken pox vaccines.

- inactivated vaccines: These contain killed germs. The various forms of influenza (flu) vaccines are of this type.
- toxoid vaccines: These contain toxins (or poisons) from the germs that have been made harmless. This type includes diphtheria and tetanus vaccines.
- component vaccines: These contain parts of the whole germ. Examples of this type are the hepatitis B vaccine, HPV vaccine, and whooping cough vaccine.

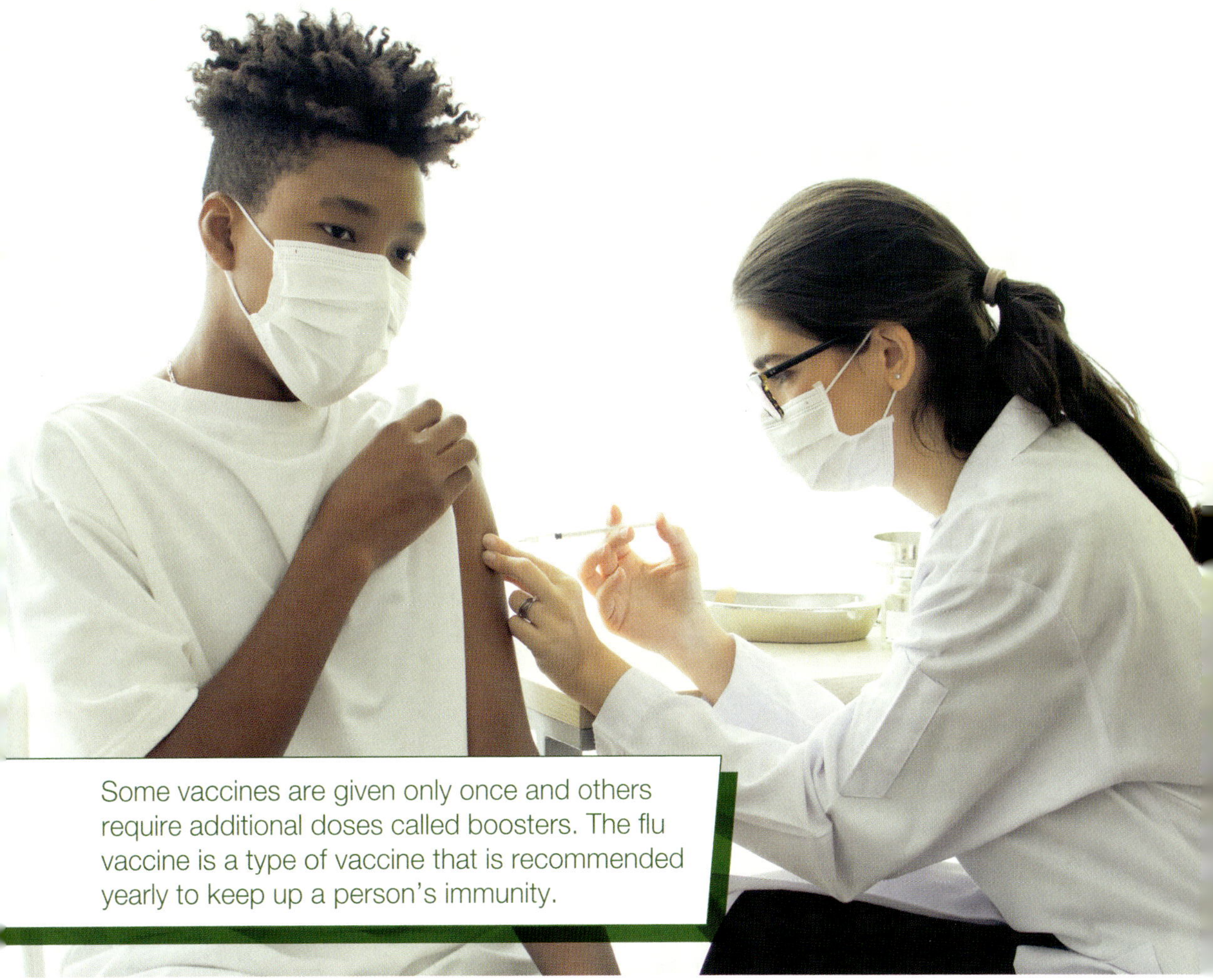

Some vaccines are given only once and others require additional doses called boosters. The flu vaccine is a type of vaccine that is recommended yearly to keep up a person's immunity.

- messenger RNA vaccines: These vaccines make proteins to trigger an immune response. This type of vaccine has been researched for decades and was approved in 2021 to protect against COVID-19.
- viral vector vaccines: These use a modified version of a different virus as a vector, or organism used to transmit a disease, to deliver protection. This has also been studied for decades for diseases such as flu, Zika, and HIV, and was approved in 2021 to protect against COVID-19.

We will probably continue to see vaccinations as the best way to deal with dangerous germs, at least in the near future. It's the most practical method we now have.

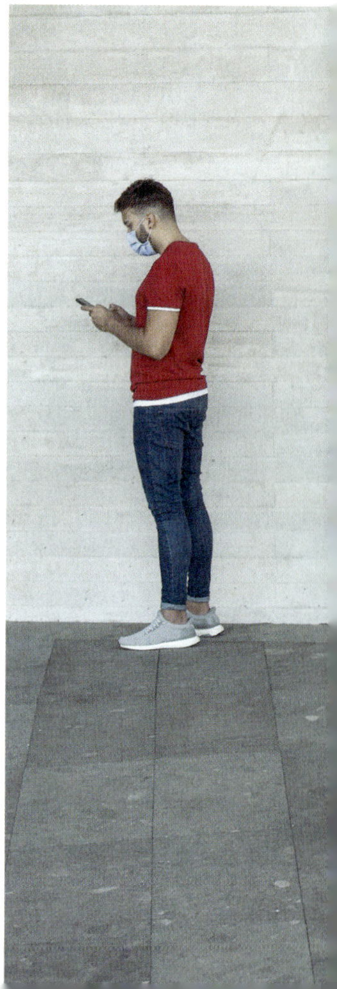

Public Health Recommendations

Public health recommendations give guidance on how to best protect ourselves when different germs pose a threat throughout the year. In 2020, the world was affected by a disease that scientists did not yet fully understand. In cases such as the COVID-19 pandemic, we took a lesson from the people who came before us. Just as populations did throughout history, we used what we knew about germs to attempt to prevent transmission and illness and adapted and changed as necessary. Public health guidelines came out regularly as medical professionals and scientists learned more about the disease.

Protective measures we hadn't previously thought of to fight against germs became commonplace. Social distancing is a public health measure we can take to try to prevent spread by simply distancing ourselves from other people. We were reminded that wearing a mask over your nose and mouth can help protect you from germs, while also protecting others from germs that may already be in your body. In addition, we were reminded of the importance of quarantining, which separates people after exposure to disease, and isolating, which separates sick people from those who are not.

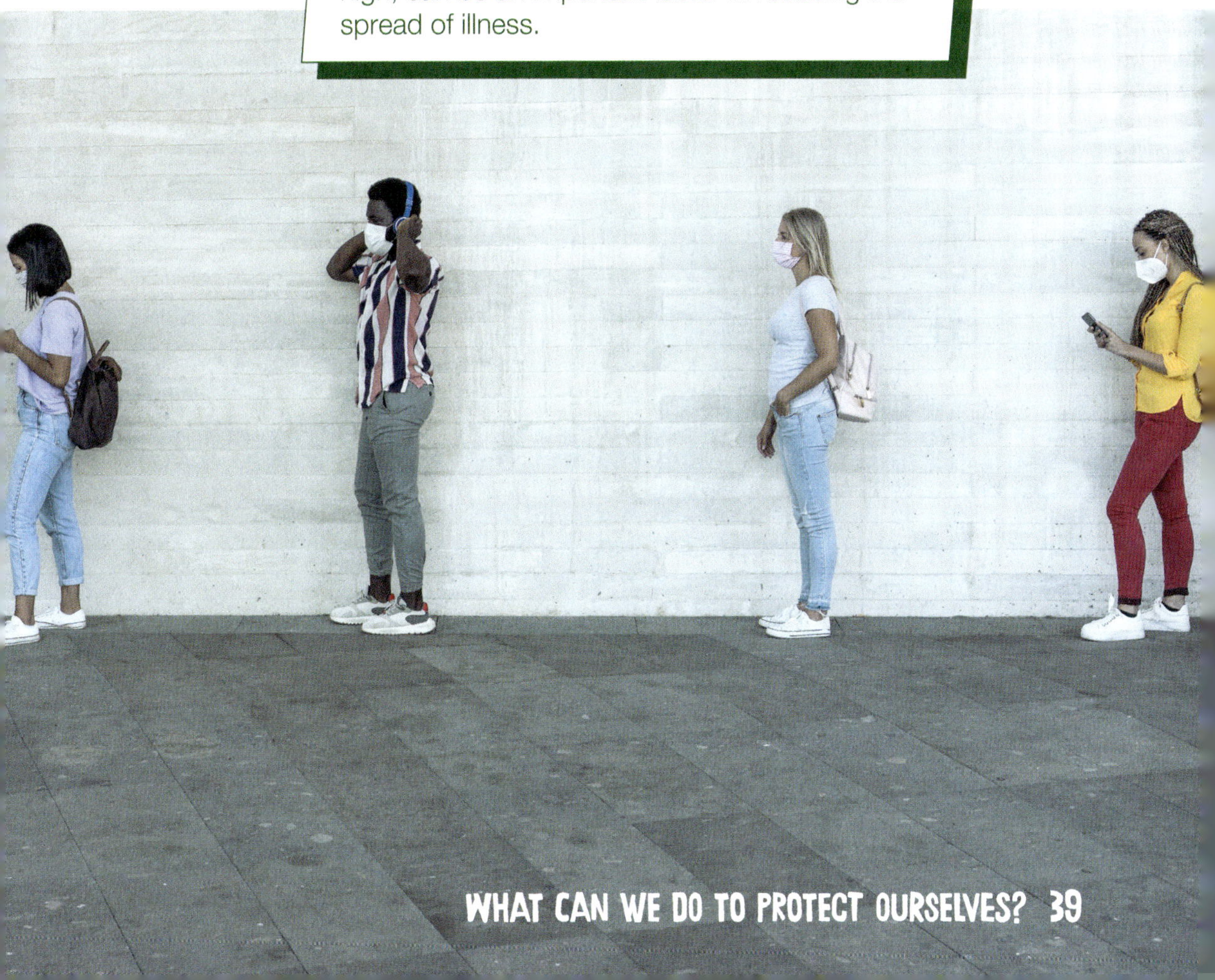

While it is sometimes difficult to remember, keeping physical distance from others, especially in situations where risk of disease transmission is high, can be an important factor in reducing the spread of illness.

PRIMARY AND PRIMORDIAL PREVENTION

You likely visit a primary care doctor every year. "Primary care" refers to a term in epidemiology called "primary prevention." The purpose of primary prevention is to prevent disease from ever occurring. When we practice safe health habits, we are participating in primary prevention to protect ourselves from germs. Getting vaccinations and keeping your body strong through exercise and good nutrition are also primary prevention strategies.

"Primordial prevention" is another term that describes strategies to keep us safe and healthy that we don't personally have control of. Think about how much harder it would be to protect yourself from germs if we didn't have sanitation systems or clean water. Primordial prevention strategies work to make sure the conditions people live in don't make it easier for them to get sick.

While definitions of these strategies are new relative to the history of germs, throughout time people have learned through observation and trial and error to use them. Today, public health professionals are dedicated to helping people understand how they can protect themselves.

These more extreme measures to protect our bodies and those around us whose immune systems may be weaker have been critical throughout the COVID-19 pandemic and have provided important lessons for any future pandemics.

The diseases that will be cured in the future are not yet known. Whether new or mutated germs will cause new problems is uncertain too. However, one thing seems certain: Germs will still be around.

They have been around throughout history, and in the future, there will still be helpful microbes and dangerous germs. There will also still be scientists who make amazing medical discoveries in the fight against disease.

WHAT DO YOU THINK?

1. What protective measures have you taken during the COVID-19 pandemic?
2. Do you think vaccines should be mandatory for everyone? Why or why not?
3. Can you think of any other ways we can stop the spread of germs?

GLOSSARY

antibiotic: A substance that can destroy or inhibit the growth of germs.

antibody: A protein made in the body that destroys or weakens germs.

antigen: Any object in the body that triggers the immune system.

antiseptic: Referring to substances or procedures (such as surgery) that are designed to ensure that infectious germs do not grow and/or are killed.

bubonic plague: A rare bacterial infection that is transmitted by fleas.

complementary: Serving to enhance or emphasize.

epidemiology: The study of the incidence, distribution, and control of diseases in a population.

humor: A substance in the body once believed by ancient scientists to determine human health.

inoculation: The introduction of a pathogen or an antigen into a living organism to help prevent disease.

lymphocyte: A type of white blood cell, the immune system's microscopic warrior against disease.

microbe: A microscopic organism, including those that can cause disease.

mucous membrane: The moist, inner lining of some organs and body cavities such as the nose, mouth, lungs, and stomach.

pandemic: A event in which a disease is prevalent all over the world and affects a significant part of the population.

sepsis: A life-threatening condition resulting from the body's extreme reaction to an infection.

treatise: A formal written article or book that deals with facts, evidence, and conclusions on a specific subject.

FIND OUT MORE

BOOKS

Denton, Michelle. *Pandemics: Deadly Disease Outbreaks*. New York, NY: Lucent Press, 2020.

Mikoley, Kate. *What Are Bacteria?* New York, NY: Gareth Stevens Publishing, 2020.

Shoals, James, and John Willis. *Immunology*. New York, NY: Smartbook Media Inc., 2021.

WEBSITES

BAM! Body and Mind
www.cdc.gov/bam/index.html
This website, run by the CDC, has information for young people about health, fitness, and social situations.

BrainPOP
brainpop.com
Watch short videos and take quizzes on science and health topics including the immune system and germs.

Nemours KidsHealth
kidshealth.org
Find doctor-reviewed health topics for kids, teens, parents, and educators along with resources to answer questions at each level.

ORGANIZATIONS

Centers for Disease Control and Prevention (CDC)
1600 Clifton Road
Atlanta, GA 30329
www.cdc.gov
The Centers for Disease Control and Prevention (CDC) is the primary U.S. government agency in charge of tracking, treating, and preventing public health threats, including infectious diseases.

National Institutes of Health (NIH)
9000 Rockville Pike
Bethesda, MD 20892
Email: NIHinfo@od.nih.gov
www.nih.gov
The National Institutes of Health (NIH) is a research facility in the Washington, D.C., area and the primary agency of the U.S. government in charge of biomedical and health-related research.

World Health Organization (WHO)
Avenue Appia 20
1211 Geneva
Switzerland
www.who.int
The World Health Organization (WHO) is the specialized agency of the United Nations primarily concerned with international public health.

Publisher's note to educators and parents: Our editors have carefully reviewed these websites to ensure that they are suitable for students. Many websites change frequently, however, and we cannot guarantee that a site's future contents will continue to meet our high standards of quality and educational value. Be advised that students should be closely supervised whenever they access the internet.

INDEX